Medical Terminology Guide for Beginners

Breakdown the Language of Medicine
- Simplified Guide -

CONTENTS

Introduction

I want to thank you and congratulate you for purchasing the book, *"Medical Terminology Guide for Beginners."* The field of medicine is quite vast. There are plenty of terms and methodologies used by medical professionals and for someone who is just starting or doesn't have a medical background; it can be really hard to figure out what all these terms mean.

Medical terminology is the universal language in the medical industry to define from human anatomy and physiology, to clinical diagnoses, procedures and processes. This language is highly applied by medical professionals to successfully communicate with each other a scientifically-based way. This language is effective as it makes communication easier. This is because it wraps various words into one. Thus, much information is conveyed in the most effective manner by doctors, nurses, and other medical professionals. Every health care professional is highly encouraged to sharpen the comprehension of medical terminology.

Medical science doesn't come with the most complex of jargons. There are a lot of simple and easy terms that you can find, and you should make it a point to get familiar with all these aspects, as it will ultimately help you to familiarize yourself with the core terminology.

Having the right kind of basic knowledge is apt for finding out more about the different medical exams and analysis that may apply to you or your loved ones. It is always good to be knowledgeable, as it helps you to be aware of what a certain diagnostic report actually means.

Sometimes, it may be that looking at the report will give you firsthand information of what the situation really is and this can help you handle your illness in an appropriate manner.

This book was written in order to help you to understand the different terminology and the details that can help you get a clearer picture of what medical reports mean. In your lifetime, you will have many examinations and will thus be presented with terminology that may not be easy for you to understand. We are going to give you directions to enhance your overall knowledge that will definitely help you out in many ways.

It includes broad alphabetical lists of root words, prefixes and suffixes, explanations, together with the terms, which are particular to parts of the body and body systems. Additionally, how to deconstruct a medical term and decode its meaning, how to pluralize, and so on will be included.
This guide will help you to:

- Comprehend the sense of medical terminology
- Comprehend, spell, and write medical terms. Apply them to communicate and record any health care situation effectively.
- Clarify the meaning of medical words to other individuals.

- Deconstruct complex words and apply the word elements to examine and establish the meaning of the medical words.
- Apply prefixes, root words, combining forms, and suffixes learned in this guide to create medical terms.

A person who has a better medical vocabulary is very lucky and particularly those who study or work in a medical ground as they use the scientific terms consistently. Some often applied medical terms in common language include, but not limited to, arthritis, hepatitis, or leukemia, where other terms are identified to be complex. Therefore, this guide will enhance you to be fluent and at the same time be able to breakdown unfamiliar and more complex words and also be able to understand them better.

So let's get started and learn medical terminology in a simplified way!

Chapter 1: The Importance of Medical Tests and Medicine

Before we talk of the different medical terminologies to help you get a clear picture of what various words truly mean, you'll need to be aware of a few more details. When you know the importance of these tests and why people opt for such examinations or even take medicines, you will be more inclined to understand the key details.

1. Health first

First of all, you need to understand that there is nothing that is more important than your health. Sometimes, you may not be aware of your declining health. It is because of the medical tests and examinations that you will be able to get a clear picture of your true condition. When you are involved in regular medical checkups, these help you to understand the state of your own health. There is no point in playing with your health and so it is vital to make sure that you discuss the results with your doctor as well as asking appropriate questions concerning anything you believe not to have been correctly explained.

2. Better medical aid

When your doctor opts for you to have different medical examinations, this takes the guesswork out of the picture and helps you get the right medical aid when needed. There are a lot of people who keep delaying examinations as they put their health on the back seat. However, you need to know that these examinations aren't useless as, in the end, it helps you know how troubled your state of health is. Your medical results will give you an idea of your health, and this will help you find out the right method of treatment that has to be taken. It's better to be informed than to avoid checkups your doctor advises you to take.

3. Routine checkups are good for you

You do not necessarily need to be ill or suffering from some kind of medical complications in order to go for health checkups. Ideally, you should make it a habit of opting for routine checkups from time to time. This is important as it can help you know in advance if there is some kind of problem that may possibly occur.

In a busy world like ours, where people are so busy doing so many things, it can be extremely hard for them to get a clear idea of how they are feeling. Furthermore, there are plenty of medical illnesses that take a lot of time to show their symptoms. So, in such cases, it is important for you to go for routine checkups at regular intervals. It might end up making all the difference. If breast cancer, for example, is found early, it can make a difference to the prognosis.

4. Reduced healthcare cost

We all know how hard it is for people to bear the costs associated with purchasing medicine. The cost of healthcare and the medical bills can be a bit too much. In such cases, if you want to cut down on the total expenses and costs, choosing medical tests and getting diagnosed early can help you save a lot of money in the long run.

The cost of healthcare is shooting upward and if you do not get checked in a timely manner, it may end up leaving illnesses undiagnosed until the last minute and that's not the best situation to be in.

These are some of the key points of importance for medical tests and examinations. It is important that you pay attention to all of these. As these medical exams can help ensure your safety and they can improve your health, it is always advisable to go for them when they are due or when advised to by your doctor. Now that you know why these exams are important, we will shift our focus to the top terminologies and wording that you may come across.

Chapter 2: An Overview of General Medical Terminology

There are so many different diseases that exist in the world and there are millions of people who are affected by them. Everyone needs to be aware of his or her body and this is why we have decided it's best to start with the basics. Let us take a look at some of the basic tests that are often carried out and – in the next chapter, the different types of medicine that can help you out.

What does it cover?

When we talk of some of the key medical terminologies, there are a lot of points that will get covered. Here are some of the key things that will be explored in this guide.

- Abbreviations for medical diagnostics: these include tests like ECF, EEG, MRI, CT scan and more.
- Some basic and common illnesses that are likely to affect many people
- Terminologies often used in health insurances
- The medical equipment for conducting tests like BPM
- The hospital departments
- Abbreviations used in hospitals
- Basic medicinal terms
- Categories or types of medicines prescribed
- Basic human anatomy

Of course, this is not an exhaustive list and there is a lot more that can be added to this. As an individual who is not hailing from the medical field, you may not be able to understand and memorize each one of them, and it is going to take you some time before you get accustomed to it all.

You can keep adding a little information to your knowledge base every time you read something new and, slowly but surely, it will help you improve your overall understanding of this important topic.

The body systems

Now, let us take a look at the core systems present in your body. We will go through a brief overview of them, as this will help you to be sure that you know which medicines are meant for which part of the body. It helps to have a basic understanding.

The skeletal system

This forms the core framework of the body and it includes bones, axial skeleton, joints and more.

The muscular system

This forms the underlying framework that connects the bones to one another. Muscles are present almost everywhere in the body and are needed for smooth functioning of all kinds of activities.

The respiratory system

This system is mainly concerned with the process of breathing air in and out. It will include body parts like neck, pharynx, trachea, lungs, larynx and bronchi.

The endocrine system

Mainly to do with the hormones, this is an important system of the body. It would also include the thyroid, pancreas, adrenal glands, gonads and even the pituitary.

The nervous system

It is often called the central nervous system as it coordinates and controls the working of all other systems. It includes the brain along with the spinal cord and most sensitive nerves and organs as well.

The cardiovascular system

This would include the blood-pumping organ, the heart,

along with the blood and the blood vessels, too.

The reproductive system

This system - as the name suggests - has to do with the main concern of reproduction. It involves the genital organs of both males and females.

The urinary system

This system consists of various organs like the kidney, bladder, urethra, ureter, and more. They work together to filter the waste out of your body and clean your blood. It also controls the amount of water and salt that will stay in your system, as all of the impurities are filtered out.

The immune system

One of the most important systems of the human body, it keeps the body running and protected from various diseases. It consists of different components that defend the body from any foreign attack. It releases antibodies into the blood that help your body fight against an illness.

The auditory and ocular system

The auditory and ocular systems are usually grouped together as they both form a part of the sensory organ system. This consists of eyes, hearing organs, glands, as well as various bones and muscles that provide vision and hearing to the individual.

These are some of the main systems of the body. Any medical disease that occurs is likely to impact one or more of these systems. There exist many tests that affect these parts of the anatomy.

Anatomical Planes

The human body consists of various positions and planes. Just like the onion, we are also made up of layers and by peeling every layer away you might gain more understanding of your anatomy. If you would like to know more about your body, then you must have some knowledge of its anatomical positions and planes. For example, how do you know you have a pain in the heart region without knowing its anatomical position?

These terms will be of a great use to you when you visit a hospital or a diagnostic center. They are often used to provide essential pieces of information regarding a respective diagnosis, letting you decode a few details on your own. You should always know what these anatomical planes stand for, as you will be better able to understand written results:

Anterior: The term is used to depict the part of the body that is towards the front.

Deep: The part of the body that is closer to the core or center.

Lateral: The plane that is towards the side of the body.

Distal: The part that is far from the point of reference.

Posterior: The plane that consists of the back of the body.

Superficial: The part that is closer to the surface of the body.

The incorrect usage of any of these planes in a sentence can change its meaning drastically. The next time you try to define something, be very specific and know which anatomical plane you are referring to.

Membranes

Understanding the five kinds of the membrane that exist in your body is essential to sharpening your knowledge regarding medical terminology. They line the internal organs and make up a major part of your anatomy. A cavity in any membrane can cause serious damage to your body as it prevents your organs and tubes from an unforeseen rupture.

By gaining more knowledge about various kinds of membranes, you can know more about your diagnosis and consult with your doctor in a more enlightened way. The following are the major five kinds of membranes in your body:

Meninges: This consists of three tissue membranes that are connected to each other. It exists in the lining that is between the spinal cord and the brain and works as a protective cover for these organs.

Mucous Membrane: It exists in the interior walls of your organs and is also found in the lining of the tubes as well. Mucous membrane protects various respiratory, digestive, reproductive and even urinary parts of our body from wear and tear.

Synovial Membrane: These multiple membranes are composed of various connective tissues and line various joint cavities. They serve the crucial purpose of keeping the bones free to move by lubricating the joint cavities.

Serous Membrane: This membrane exists in various parts of your body – from lining the cavities and protecting them from any rupture to even keeping internal organs like your heart safe.

Cutaneous Membrane: You might be looking at your cutaneous membrane right now. It is the largest and the most significant membrane in the body and covers your entire skeletal framework – your skin.

After gaining essential information about these membranes, you would be able to understand your body in a better way. Whenever you are prescribed a medicine or even asked to go for a test, it will mainly be to deal with the disorders pertaining to any of the systems. Later, we will also discuss the different categories of medicine, as that information will help you know what the general problem is which you may be facing. Types of medicine give you an idea of the general condition your doctor is treating.

In medical science, the main trick is to follow a systematic approach. When you are all set to follow a routine and systematic method rather than trying to learn too many things together, it is going to be hard for you to handle every aspect of it. Ask your physician the necessary questions if you have doubts about what is being said.

Initially, it can be a little overwhelming and for someone who is not too interested in biology or medical science and even those who are not well versed on the human anatomy, there will be too much to know and explore.

This doesn't mean that you should not even try because you never know when you may be in need of a little medical knowledge. Sometimes, it is just the right kind of information that may end up making a difference. You may be able to save someone's life by having that information. So, in such cases, it would be wrong of you not to expand your own knowledge when it comes to the field of medicine. Taking a supplementary course in first aid will also help you to gain a better understanding of common ailments.

Chapter 3: Etymology of Medical Terms

Before we start dealing with the basic medical terminology, it is essential to understand how to decode most of the words and what their root or organic word is. After identifying the organic word, you can trace it back to its actual meaning. By practicing this technique, you would be able to understand every term and how it got its present meaning.

This might interest you and you will realize every term has a story in itself. There are a lot of words in English that trace back to the Greek or Latin language and with the study of their prefix or suffix you can devise their actual meaning. Just like any other language, you can seek the assistance of Etymology to break down your word into parts and retain this knowledge so that you can use it on various occasions without any trouble, as the rules are pretty general.

By learning the following basic three parts of any word, you can get to know specific details about its organic meaning and how you can change or alter to mean slightly different things.

1. Root word

It is used to depict the core meaning behind any term and is the foundation of a word. Thus, it is the body of the word that is attached with a prefix and a suffix to derive its exact meaning.

2. Prefix

They are used in the beginning of the word, i.e. before the root word. Prefixes are of great importance as they can depict a certain condition or the circumstances that enhance the meaning of the word.

3. Suffix

They occur after the root word and are mostly attached to the root word with the help of a combining vowel. Suffixes are used to depict information regarding a certain component of the body. When it comes to medicine, they can provide more information regarding a procedure, disease, or even a certain condition.

Additionally, you might need to know what are combining vowels and combining forms. When a vowel is used to connect a root word to another root word or a suffix, then it called a combining vowel. In medical terminology, "o" is the most commonly used combining vowel. A combining form, on the other hand, is merely a combination of the root word and the combining vowel.

Deconstructing medical terms

Now when you know how every word can be broken into different parts, you can easily decode almost every medical term. It can require hours of practice and you might need to first learn the meaning of the root words to derive a superior word from it. Use the following pattern to deconstruct your word:

1. Always start at the end. That is, your initial goal would be to identify the suffix in your word.

2. Now, determine the meaning of the suffix.

3. Move to the beginning of the word and look for a prefix. Not every word can have a prefix and you have to be careful while deriving its prefix.

4. Decode the meaning of the prefix

5. After removing the suffix and the prefix, only the root word would remain. Identify it and unravel its meaning.

6. Lastly, combine all the identified meanings together and form them into a piece of information.

Let's understand it with an example by considering the word **_Cardiomyopathy._** You might have already heard the term or could even know it's meaning, but can you figure out its prefix or root word. If we start from the end, we can easily identify the suffix as "pathy," which is a widely used suffix in medicine and stands for a disease or illness. Identifying the prefix of this word is easy. It is "cardio" which means anything related to the heart. Here, "cardi" is the prefix, which means heart and "o" is simply the combining vowel. The root word is merely "my/o" which means muscles. Thus, Cardiomyopathy stands for a diseased heart muscle.

Now, let's move to a little complex example by taking the word "Rhinorrhea." The word can be broken into two parts – "rrhea" and "Rhin/o." We started by recognizing the suffix as "rrhea", which means discharge or flow. When we move to the beginning of the word, we realize that it doesn't have any prefix. You should remember that not every word is supposed to have a prefix. This leaves us with the root word "rhin" and the combining vowel "o". The medical meaning of "rhin" is the nose. Thus, Rhinorrhea means a flow or discharge from the nose, or simply, a running nose.

Wasn't that a piece of cake? We have come up with a list of some of the most commonly used root words, prefixes and suffixes that will make your job a whole lot easier, by letting you identify the meaning of some of the widely used medical terms on the go. Try to learn the following list with utmost sincerity.

Root words

These are some of the extensively used fundamental words in Medical science. Though, while deconstructing any word, you might come across a few terms having more than one root word.

Hem or Hemat: Blood or related to blood

Chrom: Color

Cepahl: Head

Enter: Intestine

Oste: Bone

Vas: Duct or vessel

Synov: synovial joint, fluid, or membrane

Gastr: Stomach related

Derm: Skin

Phleb: vein

Thromb: Clot

My: muscle or muscular

Onych: Related to nails

Pulm: Lungs

Col: Colon

Aden: Gland

Bio: Life

Brachi: Arm

Anter: Front

Audi: Hearing

Abdomin: Abdomen

Cyt: Cell

Bronch: Bronchus

Carcin: Cancer

Hist: Tissue

Gynec: Female

Encephal: Brain

Dors: Back

Or: Mouth

Optic: Sight, related to vision

Ocul: Eye

Lapar: Abdomen

Neur: Neuron or nerve related

Ot: Ear or hearing related

Path: Disease or illness

Sept: Infection

Pulmon: Lungs or respiratory related

Pharmac: Drug

Thyr: Thyroid gland

Trich: Hairlike or hair

Thorac: Chest

Ventr: Frontal part of the body

Viscer: Internal organs of the body

Prefixes

Finding a prefix can sometimes be tough. Look for these common prefixes that are used to enhance the meaning of the root word by the addition of details like number, location, time to them.

Ec: Out

Ect: Outside

A: Absence of or without something

Peri: Surrounding

End: Within or inside

Poly: a lot, many

Ab: Away

Mon: One, single

Supra: Above

Ad: Nearby or adjacent

Trans: Through, across, or crossing something

Ante: Before, prior

Post: After or behind something

Suffixes

As stated, suffixes are attached to the end of the word and usually depict a condition, disorder or an illness. Here are a few commonly used suffixes.

Emia: Blood

Uria: Urine or related to urination

Algia: pain or sense of discomfort

Tripsy: Crushing

Centesis: Tap, puncture

Sclerosis: Hardening of something

Desis: Fusion or binding of two units

Plasty: Surgery, repair or plastic reconstruction of something

Ectomy: Surgical removal of a thing

Pexy: Surgical fixation of a unit or an organ

Graphy: Recording

By using these root words, prefixes and suffixes, you can easily derive the meaning of most of the medical terms. All you need to do is break them into various units and reconstruct them in order to derive the meaning of the word. It might seem a little complicated in the beginning, but with constant practice, you can be a pro in no time. Open your medical dictionary and start practicing to be a wizard with words.

Now when you know how to decode most of the commonly used medical terms, learn more about the different categories of medicine in the next section to expand your knowledge.

Chapter 4: The Different Categories of Medicine

When it comes to medicines, they can be classified into various broad categories. Of course, it is not possible for us to categorize all medicines into specific categories, but here is some broad classification that will be of help.

Sedatives

These medicines mainly have a high amount of sleep-inducing drugs in them. The prescribed dose is taken to make a person feel drowsy. This is important, as it will help you in multiple situations. Sedatives are not administered merely as sleeping pills. They are often a part of the painkilling process and will help you to be able to cope with pain short term.

Antibiotics

These are perhaps one of the used forms of medicines. There are a lot of medicines that fall under this category. The main aim of antibiotics is to make sure that you can handle the different bacterial infections that have invaded your body.

You will often find that antibiotics are usually given during basic medical illnesses that produce a fever as they can strengthen your body in the right manner and help you to recover.

Analgesics

These are mainly painkillers. There can be various reasons for the pain and based upon the extent of pain you are facing, you will need to use the correct dosage of analgesics. Of course, your doctor will decide this. With the appropriate amount of painkillers, you will be able to keep the pain under control. It is important to know that you should not take too many analgesics as they do have side effects. You should opt for analgesics, only if a registered medical practitioner recommends you to do so. Read the literature that comes with the medication to know if are contra indications.

Mineral and vitamin tablets

There are a lot of vitamin tablets and even minerals that are found in medicines. With these vitamin tablets, you can handle deficiencies in your body. There are a lot of people who may suffer from different kinds of vitamin deficiencies. You need to first of all find out the kind of vitamin deficiency you are suffering from. Once this analysis is done, you will be able to seek the right supplements that can help you out. Ideally, these tablets should not have side effects but, once again, you should make a decision before their consumption as to whether they are suited in your particular case. Blood tests may help you to decide what these deficiencies are.

Vaccines

While vaccines are mostly given in injection format, they can still be counted as a part of miscellaneous medicines. There are a lot of vaccines that have been developed. They can help you in treating a wide variety of problems. Some of the vaccines need to be administered at an extremely young age. There are vaccines for polio, chickenpox and many more.

Growth promoters

These are similar to vitamin supplements but they have their unique nature. Growth can be stunted owing to various reasons and these promoters can help in handling the main situation and solve the problem in an apt manner. They should never be taken without medical advice.

These are some of the broad and general categories of medicines that you need to know. Of course, under each of these categories, there will be a whole lot of sub-categories too. The right medicines can help you deal with the different troubles and it increases the chances of being sure that you can make a smooth and complete recovery. Different medicines will have varying compounds present in them. Sometimes, medicines can come with similar compounds and they might even offer you the same sort of benefits as well. However, your medical professional should prescribe them, rather than self-diagnosing.

Now that you know the main categories of medicines, we need to move further to find out details of some of the most widely used medical terms. An important point to be added is that you should give yourself time to understand each of these terms and then slowly build on the knowledge because learning too many things together may not be useful.

Chapter 5: The Basic Terms

Let us now get started with some of the basic medical terms that will help you gain a better understanding. You might already be familiar with some of these terms but you can always brush up on your knowledge. Let's get it started!

Acidosis

It is the condition in the human body when it has an excessive level of acid in the blood. Acidosis is usually caused by the dysfunction of the lungs that decreases the amount of oxygen that reaches your body parts.

Acute myocardial infarction

This is also known as the heart attack in layman terms. It is mainly caused because of the damage that is inflicted on the heart muscles all of a sudden as the blood supply to the main arteries that leads to the heart is blocked.

Addiction

This happens when the patient ends up depending too much on any specific drug or thing. It doesn't necessarily have to be drugs all the time and it can also be other substances of abuse as well. Addiction mainly refers to the dependency symptom, which the body shows towards the specific drug of abuse.

Anemia

This is a medical condition that is characterized by a relative decrease in the concentration of red blood cells that are present in the blood. In this situation, the skin color may become pale.

Ancillary Services

It is used to define various rendered services that are offered by healthcare facility apart from food and accommodation. It can consist of surgical services, laboratory tests, therapy, and so on.

Angina

This is essentially the sharp cardiac pain that is caused because of the poor supply of blood to the heart muscles. Sometimes the pain can be too severe and it can even turn out to be fatal as well.

Anorexia

Anorexia is mainly the symptom wherein people face a loss of appetite. When anorexia goes on for too long, it causes bodily systems to break down. The patient may have psychological problems, which is why he/she is depriving him/herself of food.

Antidepressant

These are drugs that are used for helping people deal with the troubles of depression. With the right anti-depressant drugs, patients can come to terms with reality and this will help them be able to cope with life.

Antiemetic

The term is used for common medicines that are given to patients to control vomiting.

Antipsychotic

These drugs are mainly used to help treat patients who are suffering from psychosis. With the right drugs, psychotic people can be brought out from their trance-like state and this can be extremely helpful too.

Apnea

The temporary pause in your breathing is called Apnea. When a baby stops breathing for more than 20 seconds, then it is called Apnea of prematurity. It is usually seen in premature babies since the part of their brain that controls breathing is not fully developed.

Appendicitis

Sometimes the appendix can become inflamed and can lead to a painful condition called appendicitis. There can be swelling and even the chance of an infection. Often surgery is required to remove the appendix if it becomes infected.

Arthritis

This is the condition that occurs when the joint is inflamed. Arthritis often leads to a very painful condition and it can even make a person limp. You will have to be sure that you can analyze the extent of arthritic pain and then look for the right kind of solution.

Asthma

This is a disease of the lungs that happens because of

multiple reasons. A lot of people suffer from asthma because of an allergic reaction. They end up coughing and are likely to suffer from breathlessness problems too.

Asphyxia

It is the condition when too little oxygen or a significantly large amount of carbon dioxide is found in the body.

Autoimmune deficiency syndrome

This is one of the most feared diseases of all time. It is commonly known as AIDS and this disease mainly means that the entire immune system has failed or is in the process of failing. Owing to the failure of the immune system, it becomes difficult for the patient to put up a resistance to bacterial and viral infections.

Bacteria

Bacteria are responsible for a lot of human illness. These are mainly tiny and microscopic organisms that can cause a lot of infection and they tend to reproduce at a fast rate, which can sometimes make it difficult to control the infection.

Beneficiary

The person who is covered by the health insurance or the one who could receive benefits from the health insurance company.

Benign

The term is used to define a tumor that is not cancer.

Bilirubin

It is the yellow pigment that is found in the blood and gives a prominent cream-colored tone to the skin if found in the body in high levels.

Blood count

It is the measure of white blood cells, red blood cells, and platelets that exist in the blood.

Blood pressure

It is the pressure that is created in arteries by the pumping of the heart. An ideal blood pressure is what a healthy body should depict. Having a low or a high blood pressure can be a symptom of several diseases and should be dealt with under a physician's care.

Blood transfusion

The term is used to depict the process of giving an extra amount blood to someone. Patients who are suffering from anemia or having a lack of blood go through blood transfusions.

Bronchitis

This is a medical condition that is caused because of the infection that arises in the lungs. Owing to the extent of infection that is caused, you will need the right kind of medicines that can help you deal with the problem.

Cancer

Cancer can be a life-threatening disease in which abnormal and unwanted cells propagate uncontrollably and destroy the healthy tissues of the body. There are different kinds of cancers that are termed according to their locations. For example, lung cancer, blood cancer, prostate cancer, breast cancer, etc.

Catheter

A catheter is a tube that is used to take away or inject any kind of fluid either to or from the body.

CDHP (Consumer Driven Health Plan)

It is the kind of health insurance plan that is often tax-deductible and can help individuals to claim insurance while saving on their taxes.

CSF (Cerebrospinal fluid)

As the name suggests, the term is used to define the fluid that flows down from the brain to the spinal cord.

Cirrhosis

This is a condition caused when the liver shrinks and becomes hard enough to impair the regular functioning of the liver. Cirrhosis can lead to a lot of problems and sometimes it can even turn out to be fatal, sometimes associated with alcoholism.

Claim

It refers to the medical bill that is sent to an insurance company and uses a standardized format.

Cognition

This is a part of the brain that has to do with higher level functioning; sophistication. It includes functions like judgment, memory, and intelligence and so on.

Concussion

This is a medical condition that occurs when you suffer a blow to the head. In such cases, the person is sometime knocked unconscious.

CVD

CVD stands for cardiovascular disease. This pertains to all the diseases that can occur that will impact the cardiac system. This is why it is important for you to be aware of some of the key CVD's and the ways in which they can be treated.

Coroner

This is mainly the position of a magistrate that has been appointed for the sake of investigating why a death has occurred. In cases where sudden death occurs and one has to make a thorough analysis of what caused the death, it is a coroner who will investigate.

Delusions

This is the state of living in a whimsical state of mind. The person who is suffering from delusions may not have the right contact with reality and requires medical attention.

Depersonalization

This is a stage where the person doesn't feel connected with the environment. They may have a hard time understanding what environment their current environment. Owing to the nature of the problem, it is possible that the person may end up suffering from a mental disorder.

Dermatitis

This is a skin disorder. There are plenty of different reasons that can lead to dermatitis and you should be sure that you handle it in an apt manner. There are many treatments available.

Detoxification

This is the process by which harmful toxins and chemicals can be eliminated from your body. You need to make sure that you are using the right minerals or substances that have the capability of cleansing the body. Based upon the kind of toxins that are present in the body, you will need to choose an apt detox process.

Diabetes

This is a disease that is caused when the sugar levels in your body rise extremely high. Diabetes is mainly caused when the level of insulin falls below a normal range. Owing to this hormonal change, the amount of blood sugar, which is present in your body, will increase. Diabetes must be monitored and treated. In milder cases, it can be treated with diet changes.

Dialysis

Dialysis is the process of cleaning unwanted substances from the blood through a membrane. Our kidneys normally perform this task. Though, when a human kidney fails, the process of cleaning blood is achieved through artificial dialysis. A dialysis machine is used to substitute the normal function of the kidney.

Dementia

Dementia is the medical condition that is mainly characterized by loss of memory. The loss can be partial or complete and it has the potential to be both temporary and permanent, as well.

DME (Durable Medical Equipment)

Physical medical equipment products that can be used time and time again, such as wheelchairs or crutches.

Dyspnea

This is the condition wherein the person experiences quite a lot of trouble in breathing. Known as shortness of breath or SOB.

ECG

Also known as an electrocardiogram, this is mainly a test that acts as an electronic recording. In this test, the activity of the heart is recorded. Based on the result that is generated, people can analyze whether they are suffering from certain heart ailments. It is a noninvasive procedure that can be completed in minutes. Often used to quickly help assess whether or not someone is having a heart attack.

ECT

Also known as an electroconvulsive theory, this method is mainly used for patients suffering from depression. With the right application of this medical treatment, the apt waves can be used and it can aid in getting rid of depression. It is often used as a last resort when medications have not helped a person. Can have lasting negative side effects.

EEG

This is also known as the electroencephalogram. This medical test is mainly done for mapping the activities of the brain. There are four different kinds of waves that are produced and based upon the nature of the waves, a lot of information can be discovered, such as seizures.

Epitasis

This is the condition that is characterized by the profuse bleeding of the nose. Bloody noses can be caused from hits to the face or spontaneous. If it does not stop bleeding on its own, medical treatment may be required.

Epilepsy

Epilepsy occurs when there are many unwanted electrical discharges that occur in the brain. These cause seizures. The body movements that happen during a seizure are involuntary.

Extubation

The process of removing a tube from lungs that has been earlier inserted to provide oxygen. The opposite of extubation is intubation.

Febrile

This is the state of suffering from a fever.

Fistula

This is the exact place where one of the organs of the body ends up leading to a weird and abnormal opening right into another organ. It can be painful.

Fractures

A fracture is a broken bone. A compound fracture is when the bone is broken so badly that it sticks through the skin. It can be extremely painful and it may take a lot of time to heal completely.

Gallstones

Gallstones are stones that form in the gallbladder. Ideally, if the size of the stone is very small, you may not need to resort to surgery. Otherwise, it becomes important to go for an operation and to either remove the stones or the gallbladder.

Gastritis

This is the condition where the inner lining of the stomach becomes inflamed and it can be accompanied with nausea, vomiting, burning and pain .

Gastroenteritis

This is one of the conditions that is mainly caused when the stomach or even the intestines becomes inflamed. This inflammation can sometimes lead to infection.

Hematemesis

When a person is suffering from a lot of vomiting is also vomiting blood. Based upon the extent of the bloody discharge, it can be an indication of serious problems.

Hematoma

This is essentially the medical term for a bruise.

Hematuria

This is the state wherein a lot of blood is passed in the urine. This can be a sign of kidney stones, infection or many other types of problem that require fast medical attention.

Hemoglobin

Hemoglobin, a component of the blood, is mainly a protein that is rich in iron. It is present in abundance in the red blood cells. Its main function is to carry oxygen to the tissues of the body.

Hemoptysis

A lot of people easily confuse it with hematemesis, which is vomiting blood. Hemoptysis is when a person is cough up blood.

Heart disease

Any kind of medical disorder that includes the heart can be categorized as heart disease.

Hernia

This is a medical condition wherein one of the parts of the body ends up protruding into another. Sometimes these require surgery to repair.

Hallucination

When a person sees or hears things that do not exist. For instance, they may hear voices talking to them inside of their head. Or see things that aren't really there. Can be seen in drug abuse, schizophrenia, etc.

Hepatitis

This is the medical condition that is mainly caused by liver inflammation. When people indulge in a lot of toxic substances and even alcohol, it can end up causing hepatitis. It is also common in IV drug abusers sharing dirty needles, having sex with an infected person, or eating food that was prepared by someone with a contagious version of hepatitis.

Hospice

This is a small hospital wherein all those who have been diagnosed with terminal illness and thereby have a limited period to live can stay. These hospice ends up being the right option for all those who know that they have limited time left to spend. Hospice care is also provided in the home to allow people with a terminal disease to die in their home. Hospice is a wonderful organization.

Hyperglycemia

In this case, the level of glucose in the blood is higher than the normal range. It's often an indication of diabetes.

Hypoglycemia

In this case, there is a deficiency of glucose in the blood.

Hypothermia

This is a medical condition that happens when the body temperature drops excessively. If the low body temperature persists or continues to drop, it can lead to death. Extreme cases require emergency medical care.

Incontinence

This is a condition that happens when the person is unable to control the action of their bladder. A person can also have bowel incontinence whereby they can't control their bowels. These people are often required to wear some sort of diaper.

Infusion

The gradual delivery of a drug or any other fluid to your body through the veins is termed an infusion.

Insomnia

This is a state wherein people are unable to sleep and it can often be one of the key causes of all possible kinds of physical ailments. Everyone needs sleep and until and unless you get the adequate amount of sleep, you will not be able to carry out regular functioning. This can be a serious condition, leading to car accidents, high blood pressure, etc.

Intravenous

This is the form of injection wherein the substance and/or chemical to be injected is forced into the vein via a needle. In some specific medical ailments, it is extremely important to offer intravenous injections, as it is the only route the medication can be administered.

Ischemia

This is the condition wherein the blood supply to a certain area has been stopped. Depending upon the area wherein the blood supply is stopped, the kind of troubles that you will face can vary. When the loss of blood supply occurs in the heart, it can lead to angina, otherwise known as chest pain. Untreated ischemia in a limb, for instance, can lead to the loss of a limb or death of tissue.

Jaundice

Caused from an excess of bilirubin in the blood from a liver disease or disorder. It can appear as discoloration of the skin and eyes. There is an excessive yellow pigment that can be found in the skin. It can also sometimes be seen in newborn babies.

Korsakoff's syndrome

This is one of the key problems that occur among those who tend to drink a lot of alcohol. Alcohol addicts will end up showing symptoms of amnesia, which is the loss of memory and even confabulation, which is essentially the act of filling in the gaps in the memory by guessing.

Mantoux test

This is essentially a kind of skin test that is done for those patients who are likely to suffer from tuberculosis. With this test, you can determine whether or not a person has been exposed to TB. The test must be "read" be a professional trained to understand how to interpret the results.

Migraine

This is a condition characterized by quite an extreme headache. This happens because some of the blood vessels in the head begin to dilate. Can be very disabling and sometimes last for days. Symptoms include headache, nausea, light sensitivity, dizziness, and fatigue.

Meningitis

This is a condition that happens when the meninges (cover of the brain) becomes inflamed. It is an acute condition, usually caused by an infection, and is an emergency that needs be treated immediately.

Morbidity

This is mainly the description of the different outcome that a disease can have.

Morphine

It is a commonly used drug that is used to reduce discomfort and pain. Interestingly, morphine does not help alleviate all pain, including the pain caused from kidney stones.

Mania

This is mainly a hyperactive state of mind wherein people experience both euphoria and restlessness. The mind is in an elated state and it is very hard to control. This is often part of a bi-polar disorder.

MRI

MRI scans provide images of our organs for a better understanding of what's going on inside the body. MRI stands for Magnetic Resonance Imaging and uses magnetic fields and radio wave energies to see pictures of our interiors.

Munchausen syndrome

This is mainly a kind of syndrome that happens when someone tries to fake a medical illness so that they can seek attention. This is a psychological illness. Many of these people go to great lengths to harm themselves for attention.

Neuritis

This is mainly the state wherein the neural tissue has been inflamed and it can be extremely painful.

Nebulizer

This is a device that is controlled by an air pump. The work of the pump is to convert the liquid into a mist that can then be used for inhalation. Nebulizers work great for all those who are suffering from asthma, allergies and other breathing disorders.

Night sweats

While a lot of people tend to ignore this condition, night sweats can be an indication of several serious diseases such as cancer. It can also be caused by menopause, thyroid problems, etc. It is a common symptom of tuberculosis.

Edema

This is a state which has been characterized be the presence of fluids in the tissues. For instance, heart failure can cause swelling of the ankles, otherwise known as edema in the ankles and lower legs.

Esophagus

This is a part of the digestive tract. It is a muscular tube that runs from the mouth to the stomach. It is possible to experience esophageal spasms, which can mimic a heart attack.

Palpitations

This is a condition that occurs when the heart suddenly beats a lot faster. It does not necessarily mean a serious heart condition, but can be uncomfortable, unsettling, and worrisome. It is important to have any unusual occurrences with the heart checked by a medical professional.

Pancreas

A gland located right behind the stomach. The main purpose of the pancreas is to produce insulin. It plays a role in digestion and works in conjunction with the liver.

Paralysis

Paralysis occurs when one part of the body fails to respond. Mostly, nerve damage that can lead to paralysis. Paralysis can be temporary or permanent based on the cause.

Paranoia

This is often related to a psychological disorder like schizophrenia. It ends up leading to problems of hallucination and even delusion and other fears. Paranoia tends to trigger phobias, too and when the level of fear shoots too high, it is likely to lead to social issues as well.

PCP (Primary Care Physician)

Stands for the primary physician who would provide initial healthcare to a patient. PCP coordinates with specialists and other providers on behalf of the patient. Many health insurance companies require that person have a primary care physician to coordinate their care.

Personality disorder

This is a behavioral disease wherein the person can experience varying moods and mood swings. These include borderline personality disorder, narcissist personality disorder and histrionic personality disorder, just to name a few.

Pediculosis

When the skin gets infected by a pediculosis louse. In layman's terms, it is known as scabies. The skin becomes very itchy and the need to scratch and touch is incredibly high. It requires fast treatment as it can rapidly spread over the whole body and can also spread to other people.

Phlebitis

This is a medical condition that is characterized by inflammation of the walls a vein. Can sometimes be caused where an IV has been started, or from drug addicts using dirty needles.

Psychosis

In this condition, the person may not be in his or her "right mind" and can commit acts and deeds they may not be aware of. Their sense of judgment and memory is severely impacted. Those who are suffering from psychosis should seek immediate medical attention as this problem can worsen quickly in a very short span of time. Sometimes people in a psychotic state commit violent crimes.

Psychosomatic

Means the mind and body. This is a psychological disorder that creates physical symptoms. The mind creates problems within the body. The person experiencing the physical problems really is having the health problem. They are not "making them up" but the symptoms are caused from stress, not a virus or other illness.

Pulmonary

The word is associated with anything that is related to either the respiratory system or the lungs.

Pulse

One of the most common medical terms, it is used to define the rhythmic movement of the artery. Since the human pulse can be felt, it is the first thing that is checked by paramedics and doctors to determine the condition of the patient. It is also closely related to our blood pressure. It is usually checked and counted at the wrist or neck.

Radiology

Radiology deals with X-Rays, CT scan, MRI Scans, and other techniques that use radio and electromagnetic techniques to take detailed pictures of the inside of the body.

Rapport

It is a commonly used colloquial term, though it has a different a meaning when it comes to medicine. Often an emphatic relationship is formed between a health care worker (doctor, nurse, etc.) and the patient, which is termed as having a rapport with a patient.

Resuscitation

It is the act of reviving someone from the state of unconsciousness or even death. The term is commonly associated with CPR. It is used to define the act of taking extra measures in order to keep a patient alive. Some people do not want to be resuscitated and will sign a DNR (Do Not Resuscitate) statement to keep on file with their doctor or before a major surgery.

Scabies

This term is used to indicate an inflammatory skin condition that usually occurs due to pediculosis louse.

Schizophrenia

Schizophrenia is a mental illness. Scientists have yet to discover the exact cause of it, but it is commonly accepted at this time that schizophrenia is caused by a genetic disorder and is usually characterized by strange social behavior and thoughts. People suffering from schizophrenia often see or hear things that are not real.

Sepsis

It is used to denote a specific kind of infection, usually caused by bacteria that enter in the bloodstream and spread throughout the body. A patient is often called **Septic** when the infection has spread via the bloodstream to their entire body. Often, this is fatal.

Shock

When the body has abnormally low blood pressure due to sudden blood loss from trauma, etc. Shock is a medical term. Many lay people use the term "shock" to mean devastated. The medical term shock is an emergency and is life threatening. The laymen's term is an emotional state that is not life threatening.

Sinus

The word can have multiple meanings. It means recess, channel, or hole. The most commonly known one are the facial sinuses, which refer to a cavity in the skull bone.

Spleen

This organ is located in the upper abdominal part of the body and is an integral part of our immune system.

Sternum

It is used to depict the middle chest bone and the part in our body where ribs from each side of the chest meet. It helps protect the heart and lungs.

Steroid

The term was originally used to depict a range of chemically rich substances that are manufactured by our adrenal glands. These days, steroids are given to patients for their fast action and ability to treat inflammation. Anabolic steroids, used by athletes, are a different type of steroid used to gain muscle and weight.

Stroke

It is the condition that takes place when blood flow to the brain is blocked. Often caused by a blood clot. Symptoms include weakness, paralysis, and in severe cases even death.

Syndrome

When a collection of symptoms occur at the same time or together without a known cause. Not to be confused with a **disease**, which when a collection of symptoms occur together that do have a known cause or predictable course.

Tetanus

Tetanus is a bacterial infection that is often stimulated by a puncture wound. A vaccine is available to prevent tetanus. If not prevented, tetanus infection can often lead to death.

Thiamine

The term is synonymous to Vitamin B1, which is vital for our heart and brain. It is important to note that low levels of thiamine are often found in alcohols.

Tolerance

The medical meaning of tolerance is a process where the human body adapts to the changes made by an external force or a foreign body. After regular exposure to a substance, the body begins to need more and more of the substance in order to fulfill the desired effect.

Transference

It is the unconscious tendency of transferring one's attitude or feelings towards someone else. In psychoanalysis, it is used to depict a phenomenon where patients redirect their feelings to their therapists that were originally felt by them in the past.

Tuberculosis

A bacterial infection often referred to as TB. Usually attacks the lungs but effect any part of the body. Includes latent TB and active TB. A person with active TB is contagious. Often spread through water droplets in the air from the person coughing.

Ulcer

An ulcer is an open sore or wound that can occur on the skin or internally. The most common places ulcerations occur are the stomach lining, skin, and cornea.

Urological

The term is used to depict anything that is related to kidneys, bladder, or the urinary system.

Ventilator

It is an artificial respiratory machine that provides assistance for patients to breathe. It requires that the patient be intubated, which means that a tube is placed either through the nose or mouth, down the back of the throat to the trachea so that air can be forced into the patients lungs.

Virus

A virus is a kind of microorganism that is smaller than bacteria. It requires a host (a human cell) to reproduce. Since a virus is not destroyed by antibiotics, the infective particles can cause significant damage to the body. Some of the deadliest viruses are Ebola virus, Marburg virus, HIV, Hantavirus, Influenza, and more. All these viruses have collectively taken millions of lives to date.

Wheeze

It depicts a form of breathing that is usually accompanied with a whistling sound. It is commonly observed in asthma patients, but can also be heard from patients the chronic obstructive lung diseases, etc.

There are plenty of medical terms that are used by doctors and scientists all over the world. Though, the above-mentioned basic terms will allow you gain adequate knowledge of medicine, letting you discover more about your body will certainly help you to communicate with your doctor in a better way. Try to know the meaning of all these basic terms, and keep gaining more knowledge with ongoing research. You can become a pro in no time!

Chapter 6: Medical Terms of Body Systems

When practicing medicine or when getting medical treatment, the people concerned need to understand the terminologies used in the medical field. Medical practitioners do not, of course, have a problem with this, but laymen may have problems comprehending what their doctors mean when they write reports on them. As such, it is good to have some basic knowledge of your body and the medical language often used to refer to each part.

So, how about learning medical terms under specified categories? That could make it relatively easy for anyone to remember them, because there is, obviously, something to associate them with. First of all, the human body is made up of many organs, none of which can operate on its own. As such, different organs work together to accomplish specific functions of the body. It is such sets of organs that are referred to as body systems, and each of them is responsible for an important body function. Human beings have generally eight body systems, namely, the respiratory system; the nervous system; the digestive system; the excretory system; the endocrine system; the skeletal as well as muscular system; the circulatory system; and also the integumentary system.

In this chapter, the terms to be discussed are mostly associated with sub-systems falling under these broad body systems. As such, it is a good idea to mention what the individual body parts are that fall under the broad body systems, and also what their functions are.

Here are body systems, organs that form them, and their respective functions:

The Respiratory System

The human respiratory system comprises the lungs and nasal passages; the bronchi and the pharynx; the trachea and the diaphragm; as well as the bronchial tubes. This set of seven organs is in charge of taking in oxygen and then removing the carbon dioxide produced out of the body.

The Nervous System

The organs making up the nervous system include the brain and the spinal cord; the nerves, the eyes, nose and ears; and also the tongue and the skin; and together they are in charge of how the body conducts its activities as well as how it reacts to stimuli.

The Digestive System

The organs comprising the digestive system include the teeth and tongue; esophagus and stomach; the pancreas, liver and the intestines. They all work together as a system to break down food and absorb it so that it can be utilized by the body.

The Excretory System

The excretory system comprises the ureter, kidneys and the bladder, and also the skin. This system helps in controlling and maintaining the balance of water and salt in the body.

The Endocrine System

The endocrine system comprises the pituitary and adrenal glands; and also the thyroid gland and the gonads. This is the system whose organs produce and regulate body hormones.

The Skeletal and Muscular System

This body system is made up of the bones and body muscles, and it is in charge of all body movements as well as protection.

The Circulatory System

The circulatory system comprises the heart and the entire

lymph system, the blood vessels and the blood itself. It is in charge of transporting nutrients, water and salts all over the body, and also transporting metabolic waste for excretion. It is also plays a major role in handling cells meant to fight disease.

The Integumentary System

This comprises the entire body skin. One of its major roles is maintaining moisture within body tissue. It also regulates a person's body heat. It is also the body system that holds receptors that respond to stimuli. The integumentary system also protects the body from external injury as well as from bacteria and other disease causing microorganisms.

Appendicular Skeleton

The appendicular skeleton is a body system comprising 126 bones in total, essentially from the human upper and lower limbs, as well as the pectoral and pelvic girdle. For better visualization, the upper limb comprises the hand, wrist, forearm and the arm itself; while the pectoral girdle is the point at which the upper limb gets attached to the body.

The appendicular system is the one that enables a person to move about, protects the reproductive system, the digestive system, as well as the urinary system.

Carpel

Carpel is the body system comprising the eight tiny bones making up the wrist. The term, carpel, is derived from the word that means 'wrist' in Latin, *carpus*, as well as its equivalent in Greek, *karpós*.

Cervical Spine

This body system is made up of bony rings, seven in number, and it is to be found within the neck, somewhere between the bottom of the skull and the part of the trunk that hosts the thoracic vertebrae. They can be described aptly as the initial seven vertebrae of the human spine. The cervical spine is the thinnest and also most delicate part of the spinal column, but it still supports the head and protects the spinal cord. It is also the body system that facilitates mobility of the head and also the neck.

Coccyx

This is the body system that supports the end of the vertebrae. It is essentially a tiny bone of a triangular shape, which sits at the bottom of the human spinal column. It is basically made up of vestigial vertebrae well fused, and is commonly referred to as the tailbone.

Diarthrosis

This comprises an entire joint that moves freely, the bony part being enclosed within one articular capsule.

Femoral Neck

This passes for the femur neck, the upper section of the femur that fits well into the acetabulum. It has a flattened but pyramidal look, and it connects the head of the femur with its shaft.

Femur

This is commonly referred to as the thighbone, and it is essentially the upper part of the limb that articulates at the hip and knee.

Fibula

This is a bone on the lower leg, one of two bones found between a person's knee and the ankle. Of the two bones, fibula is the smaller one, and it lies parallel to the other bone, the tibia.

Humerus

This makes up the bone on the upper part of the arm, one that also forms the shoulder as well as elbow joints.

Lumbar Spine

This is a body system comprising vertebral bodies, five in number and making part of the human spine. These vertebral bodies happen to be stacked each on another, and with a disc fitted in between. The whole system runs from what is commonly known as the chest, technically the lower part of the thoracic spine, to the lowest end of the spine, what is known as the sacrum.

Metacarpal

This refers to each of the bones, which are five in number, which form part of the hand. In ordinary language, metacarpal is simply the human hand.

Metatarsal

This refers to each of the bones forming part of the foot. In ordinary language, metatarsal is simply taken to mean the foot, or the *metatarsus*.

Olecranon

This is the body system making the end of the ulna on the upper side, the ulna being a large bone within the forearm. It is actually the bony part that gives the elbow prominence. Ordinarily, one sees the olecranon as simply the elbow.

Patella

This is the part of the body that forms the kneecap.

Pelvic girdle

This is the body system that provides an attachment area for the pelvic fins. It is essentially the structure the human pelvis forms, enclosing some sensitive areas of the body.

Phalanges

These are the bones of a human toe or finger. This body system also passes for the phalanx. Generally when people speak of phalanges they are thinking of fingers and toes.

Radius

This forms a bone within the forearm, the forearm having two bones and the radius being the shorter one. The radius is also thicker than the other bone and is aligned to the side of the thumb.

Ribs

This is a body system comprising a series of bones that are both slender and curved. These bones are articulated to the human spine in pairs. The bones that make up the ribs are twelve in number, and they mainly protect the thoracic cavity and all the organs that lie within. The ribs run from up the thoracic vertebrae extending towards the ventral part of the body trunk, and they effectively form the main part of what is termed the thoracic skeleton. The manner in which the ribs are organized is seven pairs of them running along the front and back side of the body; three of them attached to the posterior; and two of them appearing incomplete.

Sacrum

The sacrum is made of fused vertebrae and generally lies on the lower side of the lumbar spine. It is the body system comprising a flat bone that is triangular in shape, and which lies on the lower part of the human back, right between the hipbones within the pelvis.

Shoulder Girdle

The shoulder girdle is also referred to as the pectoral girdle. It is the body system made up of a set of bones, the clavicle and the scapula, connecting the human arm and the axial skeleton.

Sternum

The breastbone is essentially what makes up the sternum.

Tarsal

The tarsal is a bone within the tarsus, the tarsus being a group of bones which are small in size and which together constitute the major part of the hind limb. A human tarsus has seven bones forming the ankle as well as the upper side of the foot. These bones are specifically three cuneiform bones; the talus; the cuboid; the calcaneus; and finally the navicular.

Thoracic Spine

This body system is essentially the central region of the spine, lying right below the human cervical spine. It consists of vertebral bodies that are twelve in number and is somewhat C-shaped.

Tibia

This body system lies between the human knee and ankle, and is one of two bones forming the main part of the lower leg. The tibia lies beneath the other bone, the fibula, and is the larger one. Both bones run parallel to each other.

Ulna

This is one of the two bones that make up the main part of the forearm, the ulna being the thinner one and also longer. It lies on the opposite side of the human thumb.

Chapter 7: Medical Terms of Body Structures

In the medical field, it is not just the organs that make up body systems that you need to know, it is also important for you to understand various terminologies, some of which describe the proximity of one organ to another; proper or ill functioning of an organ; physical position of an organ; and such other terms that touch on the medical condition of various parts of the body.

Here are some medical terms relating to the human body structure:

ab-

This is a prefix used on various parts of the body to signify away from. It could also mean off that particular part or from it.

For instance:

Abduction: You could use the term abduction when describing the act of a limb moving away from the main body

Abnormal: This is a term constantly used to indicate that what is happening is getting away from, or deviating from the normal.

Abd

This is an abbreviation which, in the medical field, is used to stand for the abdomen.

Abdomin or abdomino

Either of these terms simply stands for the abdomen.

Abdominal

The term, *abdominal*, is used in the medical field to describe something that pertains to the abdomen.

Abdominopelvic

This term is used to describe an entire body cavity that is a combination of the abdominal cavity and the body's pelvic cavity. The organs found within this large body cavity include a good part of the small intestines as well as the large intestines; the liver and pancreas; the spleen and the stomach; and also the kidneys plus the gallbladder.

Abduction

This term signifies moving away from the main body

Adduction

Adduction carries the notion of moving towards the main body

Adhesion

Adhesion in the medical sense is the forming of scar tissue that looks like a band, which in the process binds surfaces of the anatomy that are ordinarily separate.

Adjective endings:
ac/al/ar/ary/eal/ic/iac/ior/ous/tic

These suffixes that are used to form adjectives denote *pertaining to*.

Here are some simple examples:

Abdominal	Myalgia	Bacteriocidal	Oesophageal	Hepatic artery
Femoral	Biliary tract	Corneal	Perineal	Hematotic

-ad and ad-

When used in a medical sense, the suffix and prefix carry the meaning of *towards* or *in the direction of*. For example:

- medi-ad stands for *towards the center* or the *middle*
- ad-duction stands for movement of a body part towards the middle part of the main body.

Anastomosis

Anastomosis is used to refer to the joining of two blood vessels or two ducts through a surgical procedure, so that the blood can pass freely from one side to the other. The term is also used when the surgical procedure is done to connect different segments of the bowel to facilitate smooth flow of bowel content.

Anatomical position

This is a term used to describe a standing position, where the whole body is upright and head is held facing upwards, then the arms are placed on the sides of the body with palms facing forward. In this anatomical position, the legs are parallel to each other while the feet stand slightly parted with the toes pointing in front.

Ant

Ant, in the medical field, is an abbreviation standing for *anterior.*

anter/ior

This term is used to describe the position of a body structure or a body organ, when it appears on the front side of the body.

anter/o

This term refers to the body front. In some instances the term *anterior* may stand in for it.

AP

AP, in the medical arena, stands for anteroposterior

Back

Back in the medical language refers to the posterior side of the body or the behind

Bx

Bx is used to denote biopsy

Cartilage

The cartilage is a term referring to the ribs

Caud(ad)

This term is used to denote in the direction of the tail or the posterior. From the term, an adjective is derived – caudally.

Caudo

Caudo is simply the tail or the lower side of the human body, and in many instances it is used as a form of prefix or even suffix.

For example:

- Caudofemoralis – this term representing a muscle within the pelvic limb. It is derived from the Latin word, *cauda*, which means thighbone.

- Craniocaudal – this term indicating the direction taken by an X-ray beam to penetrate the body. In medical use, the point of entry of the X-ray beam is termed the *cranial* end, while the point at which the beam exits the body part under examination is referred to as the *caudal* end.

Cauterize

This is a term used to indicate the process of burning tissue that is found to be abnormal, using a range of options including heat, electricity, and even chemicals like silver nitrate. Sometimes the abnormal tissue is destroyed by freezing, and the term, *cauterize*, still applies.

cephal/o

This term is used to refer to the head. From the term, *cephalad* is then derived, and it means towards, or in the direction of, the head.

cervic/o

This is a term used to refer to the human neck. There are other terms derived from it like *cervix uteri*, which means the uterus' neck

Cervical

Cervical, is a term used to mean that which pertains to the human neck. It can also be used to mean that which pertains to the uterus' neck

chondr/o

This is a term used to mean cartilage, a name derived from the Greek language where *chondros* means cartilage.

chondr/oma

This refers to a mass of cartilage cells that have grown like a tumor. Sometimes it is actually a tumor. Sometimes this mass of tumor like cells develops on a cartilage surface and other times it develops on the inside only to gradually emerge from the medullary cavity's cartilage.

CT

CT stands for computed tomography

Crani(o)

This is a term used to refer to the human skull, otherwise known as the cranium.

Cranial

Cranial means that which pertains to the human skull or to the cranium.

CXR

CXR is an abbreviated way of saying, chest X-ray, and it can also mean chest radiograph.

Cyt(o)

This is a term for a cell. It is often used as a prefix to form terms like cytoplasm, cytokinesis and such others showing some relationship with cells.

Cytology

In medicine, this term refers to the study of human cells.

Cyt-o-lysis

This is a term that means cell separation, cell dissolution or even cell destruction. It comes from the combination of the term denoting cell, cyto, and *–lysis*, where *–lysis* means loosening, separation, or even destruction.

cyt/o/meter

This is a name given to an instrument used to count or measure cells. It is of standard specifications and comprises a glass chamber whose volume is clearly known. It may also comprise a glass slide that is well ruled.

Cyto-toxic

This is a term used to refer to a substance that is capable of destroying cells. *Toxic* on its own stands for poison, and of course, *cyto* is used in reference to cells.

Dist/al

This term refers to some point very far from the central area or from the main body. It is often used in contrast to what would be considered *proximal.* Proximal is the term used to mean close to the center of the main body or close to the point at which the organ is attached to the main body.

Dist(o)

This is a term used to denote farthest or just far.

Doppler

This refers in connection to technology that works with sound waves of ultra high frequency to produce audible blood flow sounds as blood runs through the arteries. The technology used is what is called Doppler technology.

Dors(al)

This is used to indicate that something has something to do with the body's posterior or the back of it. One can, for instance, speak of the *dorsal* view.

Dors(o)

This is a term referring to the back of the human body and often serves as a prefix. A good example is the term, dorsolateral, which bears the meaning of relating to someone's back.

Endoscopy

This is the process where someone uses an endoscope, which is a lighted instrument of a specialized nature, to visually examine the inside of a body organ or a cavity.

Epigastric region

This refers to a person's area above the stomach or actually on it.

Fluoroscopy

This is a radiographic procedure that shows an organ's internal movement through imaging done by X-ray. It makes use of a fluorescent screen as opposed to a photographic plate, and ends up producing vivid visual images of a person's inside.

Frontal plane

This is a term used the same way coronal plane is used. It is that part of the body marking the section where the human body is divided into two equal parts, one being the body front or the anterior, and the other being the back or the posterior. The front part of the body and the back are also termed the ventral and dorsal respectively.

Gastr(o)

This is a term given to the stomach.

Gastric

Gastric is a term used to mean that something pertains to the stomach.

Inguin(o)

This is a term that refers to the groin.

Inguinal

Inguinal is a term used to mean that which pertains to the groin

Hist(o)

This is a term used to mean body tissue, and it is often used as a prefix to indicate something pertaining to tissue.

Histologist

A histologist is an expert who has studied matters pertaining to body tissue.

Traverse plane

This term is used to refer to a horizontal plane, which can also be cross sectional. It divides the body into the upper and lower part, which are seen as the superior and inferior sections respectively.

Hypochondriac region

This is the section of the body that lies immediately below a person's ribs.

Hypogastric region

This term is used to refer to the section of the body immediately below a person's stomach.

Ili/o

This is a term used to refer to the ilium. It can also mean flank. It is sometimes used to form compound words that have something to do with the ileum.

Good examples:

iliofemoral	iliolumbar	iliocostal	iliocolotomy	Iliocaudal muscle
iliothoracopagus	ilioxiphopagus	iliocostalis	iliopagus	iliococcygeal

Iliac

This term is used in the medical field to denote that something pertains to the ilium.

Ilium

This is the upper part of the hipbone. It also carries the meaning of the area within the abdomen, extending from the place where ribs end to the groin or the pubic area.

Infer(ior)

This is a term used in the medical field to indicate that the area is somewhere below or towards the end or tail.

Infer(o)

This term simply means a place below or somewhere lower than another.

Inflammation

This is the response the body produces as protection when it is exposed to an allergy or irritation of sorts, or even an infection.

Inguin(o)

This is a term used to refer to the groin.

Lat

In the medical field, *Lat* denotes lateral.

Lateral

As for lateral, it simply means something that pertains to, or associated with, the side

Later(o)

This term denotes leaning towards one side. Sometimes it is also used to denote *side*

LLQ

People in the medical field use LLQ as stand for *Left Lower Quadrant*

Loins

Loins is a term that covers the area of the body representing the lower back

Lumb(o)

The term lumb, and sometimes lumbo, is used to refer to the loins or lower back

Lumbar

This is another term that people in the medical field use to show that something pertains to or is linked to the area of the loins or the lower back.

The lumbar region

The lumbar region is that area of the human body just below the loins or just below the lower back.

LUQ

These letters make an abbreviation for Left Upper Quadrant

MRI

These letters make an abbreviation for Magnetic Resonance Imaging

Medi(ad)

This term refers to an area towards the center or the middle. It is derived from Latin where it simply means *middle*. It is often used to make up other words denoting middle position, such as median; medium; mediator; and such others.

Medi(al)

This is a term used to denote that which pertains to the center or the middle

Medi(o)

This term means middle. It is often used to form other words in the medical field such as mediotarsal.

Median plane

The median plane is also referred to as the midsagittal plane. This is the area of the body that divides the human body in a symmetrical manner, right from the top to bottom. In effect, the median plane divides the human body laterally into two parts that are equal and similar – the left side and the right side.

Nucle(ar)

This is a term that indicates something has something to do with the nucleus

Nucle(o)

This refers to the nucleus, the spheroid body that is found inside a cell. It is enclosed within a double membrane, which is often referred to as nuclear envelop. Whatever is contained in this spheroid body, including chromosomes, is referred to as nucleoplasm.

Nuclear scan

This is a process applied as a diagnostic technique, where some radiopharmaceutical is introduced into the body by way of ingestion, inhalation or even injection, and then an image is produced of the organ or part of the body being checked, as the concentration of the radiopharmaceutical is recorded.

PA

These letters are used to form an abbreviation used variously in the medical field. Some of its meanings include pernicious anemia; posteroanterior; pulmonary artery; or even Physician Assistant.

Pelv(i)

This term can be substituted for pelv(o), and what each of them means is pelvis.

Pelvimeter

This term refers to an instrument that medical practitioners use to measure the size of the pelvis.

Periumbilical

This term is used to mean something that relates to the area near the umbilicus.

PET

These letters make up the abbreviation Position Emission Tomography

Positron Emission Tomography

This term that is abbreviated as PET, is a radiographic technique. It combines the use of computed tomography and that of pharmaceuticals, to show the parts of the body that are metabolizing the radiopharmaceuticals, and those that are fall short in metabolism.

Poster(ior)

This term is used to refer to something that pertains to the part of the body near the rear. It is sometimes called the caudal end.

Proxim/o

This is a term used to refer to an area that is close to the body center or a place close to the reference point.

Radiography

This is the term given to the process where ionizing radiation is sent to penetrate the body from an external source, enabling the production of shadow images which have been captured, onto a photographic film.

Radiopharmaceutical

This term refers to a drug that bears radioactive material meant to penetrate a part of the body in the process of scanning.

RLQ

These are letters that mean Right Lower Quadrant

RUQ

These are letters standing for the Right Upper Quadrant

Scan

Scan is a technique used in the medical field to record and display an image of a part of the body, an organ, or even an entire system, for the purpose of studying it.

Sepsis

The term, sepsis, refers to the way a body responds by way of inflammation when it is infected, and when the situation is such that the person is experiencing fever and has low blood pressure; and also when the heart rate is elevated and the respiratory rate too.

Single-Photon Emission Computed Tomography

This term is abbreviated as SPECT. It is a form of nuclear imaging where some radioactive tracer is injected into the body to enable scanning of a chosen organ of the body with the intention of studying it. The technique makes use of a specialized type of gamma camera, to detect any emitted radiation, and to produce an image that is 3-dimensional, and that from a varied range of views.

SPECT

SPECT is used in the medical field as abbreviation for Single Photon Emission Computed Tomography.

Spin(o)

This is the term used in the medical field to refer to the spine of the human body

Spinal

The term, *spinal*, is used to denote something that has something to do with the spine or the spinal column in general.

Super(o)

This is a term used to mean upper part or some part above

Superior

Superior is used to indicate something that pertains to some higher level or something that is above another in comparison. It is also used sometimes to mean closer to the head.

Thorac(o)

This term is used to refer to the chest.

Thoracic

This term is used in the medical field to mean something that has some association with the chest.

Tomography

This is a radiographic technique that is used to show a detailed slice of body tissue or any other part of the body, the area being of some pre-determined depth. The technique shows this cross section of body organ by producing a film.

U & L

These are letters used as abbreviations in the medical field to mean Upper and Lower. Sometimes the same abbreviation is carried as U/L

Ultrasonography

This is a term used to refer to the imaging technique applied in the medical field, to produce a good image of the inside of a body organ or body tissue. The technique makes use of ultrasound, which is essentially a mass of high frequency sound waves, bouncing off the body to produce the required image.

Umbilic(o)

This term simply means navel. Sometimes the term, *umbilicus*, is used in its place.

Umbilical region

The umbilical region is the area of the human body close to the naval.

US

This combination of letters makes up an abbreviation meaning ultrasound. Sometimes it also stands for ultrasonography.

Ventr(o)

Ventro is a term used in the medical field to mean the belly or the side of the belly.

ventr(al)

This term is used to indicate that something has some association with the belly.

Chapter 9: Formation of Plurals

Words in the medical jargon do not necessarily follow the rules of conventional language when forming plurals. In short, when changing words from singular to plural in the medical context, you should not seek to observe the rules of standard English, but rather the unique rules that apply in the medical field. As such, it is important to learn the rules that govern the change from singular to plural in the medical field. Even then, just as in standard English, there are those words that do not conform to any of the laid down rules, and so they can only be studied and put to memory in their uniqueness.

Here are various categorizations:

Medical terms ending with −a

What you need to do is drop the letter 'a' at the end, and in its place put 'ae'. A good example is *vertebra* which is singular, and which becomes *vertebrae* in its plural form. Another good example is *pleura*, a term in singular form, and which becomes *pleurae* in the plural form.

Medical terms ending with −is

What happens in this instance is that the 'is' gets dropped, and in its place an 'es' is written to form the plural form of *that* word. A good example is *arthrosis*, which is in singular, and which becomes *arthroses* in its plural form. Another good example is *diagnosis*, a medical term in singular, which becomes *diagnoses* in plural.

Other such examples include *analysis* changing to *analyses*; *exostosis* changing to *exostoses*; *metastasis* changing to *metastases*; *prognosis* changing to *prognoses*; and *testis* changing to *testes*.

Other times, the medical term may end in 'is' in singular and have its plural end in 'ides'. For example, *epididymis*, a term in singular, becomes *epididymides* in plural and *iris* becomes *irides*.

Medical terms ending with –ix or -ex

In cases like these, you need to drop the 'ix' or 'ex' as the case may be, from the singular form of the word, and then replace it with 'ices'. A good example is *appendix* which is in singular form, and which becomes *appendices* in its plural form. Another example is *fornix*, which is in singular, and which becomes *fornices* to form the plural form.

Medical terms ending with –itis

Words like these drop the 'itis' ending from their singular form, and they replace it with 'itides' to form their plural form. For example, the word *arthritis* is singular, and it becomes *athritides* in its plural form. Another good example is *hepatitis*, which is in singular, and which becomes *hepatites* in plural.

Medical terms ending with –nx

What happens in such instances, the 'nx' is dropped and substituted with 'nges'. A good example is the word *phalanx*, which is in singular, and which changes to become *phalanges* in plural. Another is the *larynx*, which is singular, but which becomes *larynges* as plural.

Medical terms ending with –um

Terms like these drop the 'um' from their singular form, and in their place, they take up 'a' to form the plural. A good example is *endocardium*, which is singular, and which becomes *endocardia* in its plural form. Another one is *myocardium* which is in singular, and which becomes *myocardial* in plural form.

Other common medical terms under this category include *acetabulum* that changes to *acetabula*; *antrum* that changes to *antra*; *atrium* that changes to *atria*; *bacterium* that changes to *bacteria*; *diverticulum* that changes to *diverticula*; *labium* that changes to *labia*; and *medium*, which becomes *media* in the plural form.

Medical terms ending with –us

In such medical terms, the 'us' is dropped from the end of the singular form of the word, and is replaced with 'i'. A good example is the word *digitus*, which is in singular, and which becomes *digiti* in the plural form. Another is oesophagus, which in plural becomes oesophagi.

Other similar medical terms include *alveolus* that changes to *alveoli*; *bronchus* that changes to *bronchi*; *coccus* that changes to *cocci*; *embolus* that changes to *emboli*; *fungus* that changes to *fungi*; *glomerulus* that changes to *glomeruli*; and *meniscus*, which changes to *menisci* in the plural form.

Some other words end in 'us' in singular, but drop it in the plural form, substituting it with 'era' and sometimes 'ora'. A good example is *viscus* which is in singular, and which becomes *viscera* in plural. Another example is the term, *corpus*, which changes to become *corpora* in plural.

Medical terms ending with −y

Such medical terms turn to plural by dropping the ending 'y' from their singular form, and replacing it with 'ies'. A good example is the word, *therapy*, which becomes *therapies* in its plural form. Another good example is *cardiomyopathy*, a medical term in its singular form, and which becomes *cardiomyopathies* in plural.

Medical terms ending with −ion

There are medical terms ending in 'ion' when in singular, but which change into plural by simply adding an 's'.A good example is the term *chorion* which is in singular. To make it plural, you simply need to add an 's' at the end of the singular form so that it becomes *chorions*.

Medical terms ending with −ma or −oma

When medical terms end in 'ma' or 'oma' in their singular form, you just need to add 'ta' to the end of that word to form its plural. Some good examples include *carcinoma* that changes to *carcinomata*; *condyloma* that changes to *condylomata*; *fibroma* that changes to *fibromata*; and *leiomyoma*, which changes to *leiomyomata* in the plural form.

Medical terms ending with −yx; -ax; or −ix

In such instances, the medical terms change in their plural form so that the 'x' at the end becomes 'c'and then takes up 'es' as an addition. Some good examples include *appendix*, which changes to *appendices*; *calyx*, which changes to *calyces*; *calix*, which changes to *calices*; and *thorax*, which changes to *thoraces* in the plural form.

Some terms used in the medical field do not follow any set format, and so you just have to know what their individual plural form is.

Here are some examples:

- *Vas*, which in the medical field is a duct facilitating the flow of blood, semen and such other body liquid, has its plural as *vasa*.

- *Pons*, a body part located between the medulla oblongata and the middle part of the brain, becomes *pontes* in plural.

- *Femur*, one of the body bones, is in singular, and it becomes *femora* in plural.

- *Cornu*, which is some bone projection in the body, is in singular, and it changes to *cornua* in the plural form.

- *Paries*, which is some cavity wall, is singular, and its plural is *parietes*.

- *Corpus*, the major part of a body organ, is in singular, and its plural is *corpora*.

- *Meatus*, which is a body opening like that in the ear, is in singular, and it does not change its form in plural; meaning its plural is still *meatus*.

- *Plexus*, which is a network of body vessels, is in singular, and its plural is *plexuses*.

- *Viscus*, which represents an internal body organ such as liver or lungs, is in singular, and its plural form is *viscera*.

Conclusion

Congratulations on your completion of this medical guide! Understanding medical terminology can get tough at times and in this guide we tried our best to include every kind of essential information to help acquaint you with common medical terms.

We are sure that with the help of our suggested method, you can now easily decode any medical term, hassle-free. Try to remember the root words, prefixes, and suffixes that we have shared here to keep up to date.

A comprehensive list of some of the most commonly used medical terms was also been created. We have tried to create an extensive list by including information related to radiology, insurance terminology, anatomy, diseases, and other widely used terms. You might have heard of a few of these terms before, but now when you know their meaning, you can certainly use them in the proper context.

Medical science has certainly come a long way in the last few years and if you want to keep yourself updated with the current trends, you'll need to the standard terms of the industry. Now, with the help of this educational book you can understand your body and various medical terms in the proper way. It will help you communicate with your doctor and you can impress the people around you with your knowledge.

You can continue to harness your skills and knowledge by continued education and reading. Take care of your body and your health. Be safe and stay fit!

60383929R00066

Made in the USA
Middletown, DE
15 August 2019